A COMPREHENSIVE GUIDE TO DEALING WITH VAGINISMUS

Unlocking the secrets of intimacy for a better sex life.

Dr. Jamie Etta.

Copyright 2023. **DR. JAMIE ETTA.**

TABLE OF CONTENTS

INTRODUCTION.

Welcome to the comprehensive guide on dealing with Vaginismus. In this guide, we will explore the various aspects of Vaginismus, including its definition, causes, prevalence, and the impact it can have on daily life. Vaginismus is a condition that affects many individuals, and understanding it is crucial for those who experience it, as well as their partners and loved ones.

Firstly, we will delve into the concept of Vaginismus, providing a clear understanding of what it is and how it manifests. We will explore the different types of Vaginismus and discuss the signs and symptoms that individuals may experience. Additionally, we will address the process of diagnosing Vaginismus and debunk common misconceptions surrounding this condition. Seeking professional help is an important step in managing Vaginismus effectively. Furthermore, we will discuss the various healthcare providers who can offer assistance, such as gynecologists, therapists, and pelvic floor physical therapists. We will also explore the benefits of support groups and online communities, providing a comprehensive overview of the available resources. Treatment options for Vaginismus will also be thoroughly examined. This will include education and counseling, pelvic floor physical therapy, the use of graduated vaginal dilators, Botox injections, and surgical options. Each treatment option will be explained in detail, allowing individuals to make informed decisions about their own care. Self-care techniques play a crucial role in managing Vaginismus and we will explore relaxation exercises, breathing techniques, pelvic floor exercises, and alternative therapies such as yoga, meditation, and acupuncture. These techniques can help individuals develop coping strategies and promote overall well-being.

Maintaining open communication and intimacy is essential for individuals with Vaginismus and their partners.

We will further discuss strategies for talking to your partner about Vaginismus, exploring non-penetrative intimacy, enhancing emotional connection, and seeking couples therapy. These approaches can help strengthen relationships and foster understanding. Coping with Vaginismus can be challenging, and this book will provide strategies for dealing with them. Building a support network and seeking professional help for mental health will also be discussed, emphasizing the importance of emotional support during the journey.

CHAPTER 1

UNDERSTANDING VAGINISMUS.

Vaginismus is a condition that affects some individuals with vaginas, causing involuntary muscle spasms in the pelvic floor muscles. These spasms can make it extremely difficult or even impossible for someone with vaginismus to engage in vaginal penetration, including sexual intercourse, using tampons, or undergoing gynecological examinations. The specific reason for vaginismus is not generally clear, yet being a blend of physical and mental factors is accepted. Some common causes include past traumatic experiences, such as sexual abuse or painful vaginal infections, as well as anxiety, fear, or negative beliefs about sex. It's important to note that vaginismus is not a conscious choice or a sign of a person's lack of desire for sex. It's worth noting that vaginismus is a treatable condition, and many individuals with vaginismus are able to overcome it and engage in pain-free vaginal penetration. Seeking professional help and support is essential for those affected by vaginismus, as it can significantly improve their quality of life and sexual well-being.

CAUSES OF VAGINISMUS. Vaginismus can have various causes, and it is often a combination of physical and psychological factors. Here are some common causes of vaginismus:

1. Psychological Factors:
Psychological factors can play a significant role in the development of vaginismus. These factors can include fear, anxiety, past traumatic experiences, negative beliefs about sex, and relationship issues.

A. Fear and anxiety: Fear of pain or discomfort during vaginal penetration can lead to muscle tension and involuntary contractions in the pelvic floor muscles. This fear can be rooted in various factors, such as previous painful experiences, medical procedures, or cultural beliefs that portray sex as painful or shameful. The anticipation of pain can trigger a protective response, causing the muscles to contract involuntarily, making penetration difficult or impossible.

B. Past traumatic experiences: Women who have experienced sexual trauma or abuse may develop vaginismus as a protective response to potential pain or discomfort. Trauma can create deep-rooted fear, anxiety, and negative associations with sexual activity, leading to involuntary muscle contractions and avoidance of vaginal penetration.

C. Negative beliefs about sex: Negative beliefs or attitudes towards sex can also contribute to the development of vaginismus. Societal taboos, cultural or religious influences, and lack of comprehensive sexual education can lead to misconceptions and anxieties about sex. These negative beliefs can create a cycle of fear, anxiety, and muscle tension, making penetration challenging.

2. Fear of Pain: The fear of pain is a common cause of vaginismus. It often stems from previous traumatic experiences, such as sexual abuse or painful medical procedures involving the genital area. These experiences can create a psychological association between vaginal penetration and pain, leading to a fear response. The fear of pain can activate the body's natural defense mechanism, causing the pelvic floor muscles to involuntarily tighten and contract. This reflexive response is an attempt to protect the body from potential harm or discomfort. However, in the case of vaginismus, it can create a cycle of anxiety and muscle tension that makes penetration difficult or impossible. Fear of pain during intercourse or other vaginal penetration can trigger the body's natural defense mechanism, causing the pelvic floor muscles to contract involuntarily. This fear can be rooted in previous painful experiences, cultural or religious beliefs, or misconceptions about sex.

3. Lack of Sexual Education:

Lack of sexual education can contribute to the development of vaginismus in several ways. Firstly, a lack of accurate information about the female reproductive system and sexual health can lead to misconceptions and misunderstandings. Without proper education, individuals may have unrealistic or incorrect beliefs about vaginal penetration, causing anxiety and fear around the act itself. This anxiety can trigger the involuntary muscle contractions associated with vaginismus.

Additionally, a lack of sexual education can result in a lack of knowledge about arousal, lubrication, and relaxation techniques. These factors are essential for comfortable and pleasurable sexual experiences. Without this knowledge, individuals may not know how to properly prepare themselves physically and mentally for vaginal penetration, increasing the likelihood of experiencing pain or discomfort.

Furthermore, societal taboos and stigmas surrounding discussions of sex and female sexuality can contribute to a lack of sexual education. These taboos may prevent individuals from seeking information or support, leading to a lack of awareness about conditions like vaginismus and the available treatment options. It is crucial to address the lack of sexual education by promoting comprehensive and inclusive sexual health education programs that provide accurate information about the female reproductive system, consent, pleasure, and communication. By increasing awareness and understanding, individuals can be better equipped to prevent and address conditions like vaginismus.

4. Relationship Issues: Difficulties within a relationship, such as poor communication, unresolved conflicts, or lack of emotional intimacy, can contribute to vaginismus. Relationship problems can create stress, anxiety, or a lack of trust, which can manifest as muscle spasms during attempted penetration. Intimate relationships are built on trust, communication, and emotional connection. When these aspects are lacking or strained, it can

lead to various problems, including sexual difficulties like Vaginismus. Here are a few ways relationship issues can contribute to Vaginismus:

A. Lack of trust or emotional safety: If there is a lack of trust or emotional safety within a relationship, it can create anxiety and fear around sexual intimacy. This anxiety can trigger the involuntary muscle contractions associated with Vaginismus.

B. Communication problems: Effective communication is crucial in any relationship, especially when it comes to discussing sexual desires, boundaries, and concerns. If communication is lacking or there are misunderstandings, it can lead to unresolved issues and anxiety, which can contribute to Vaginismus.

C. Relationship conflicts: Ongoing conflicts, unresolved arguments, or a general lack of emotional connection can create stress and tension within a relationship. This stress can manifest physically, leading to Vaginismus or exacerbating existing symptoms.

5. Physical Factors: Certain physical factors can contribute to vaginismus. These may include infections, hormonal imbalances, vaginal dryness, or structural abnormalities. In some cases, a previous medical procedure or surgery in the pelvic area can also lead to vaginismus. Here are some of the physical factors that may play a role:

A. Pelvic floor muscle dysfunction: Vaginismus can be caused by an abnormality or dysfunction in the pelvic floor muscles. These muscles may be overly sensitive or have increased tension, leading to involuntary contractions and pain during attempted penetration.

B. Trauma or injury: Physical trauma or injury to the pelvic area, such as sexual abuse, childbirth trauma, or pelvic surgery, can contribute to the development of vaginismus. These experiences can create a fear response, causing the pelvic floor muscles to contract involuntarily as a protective mechanism.

C. Infections or medical conditions: Certain infections, such as urinary tract infections or yeast infections, can cause discomfort or pain during intercourse, leading to muscle tension and vaginismus. Additionally, medical conditions like endometriosis or interstitial cystitis can contribute to pelvic pain and muscle spasms.

D. Hormonal imbalances: Hormonal imbalances, such as low estrogen levels, can lead to vaginal dryness and discomfort during intercourse. This discomfort can trigger muscle tension and spasms, contributing to vaginismus.

E. Chronic pain conditions: Individuals with chronic pain conditions, such as fibromyalgia or vulvodynia, may be more prone to developing vaginismus. The presence of ongoing pain can heighten anxiety and fear of intercourse, leading to muscle tension and involuntary contractions.

TYPES OF VAGINISMUS.

There are generally two main types of Vaginismus which includes:
1. Primary; and
2. Secondary.

1. Primary Vaginismus:
This type of Vaginismus occurs when a person has never been able to have penetrative sex or experience any form of vaginal penetration without pain or discomfort. It often starts from the very first attempt at intercourse and can persist throughout a person's life if left untreated. Primary Vaginismus is typically not related to any

specific physical condition, but rather to psychological or emotional factors, such as anxiety, fear, or trauma. The severity of primary vaginismus can vary from person to person. Some individuals may experience mild discomfort or pain during attempted penetration, while others may find any form of penetration impossible due to the intense muscle contractions. Primary vaginismus can have a significant impact on a person's sexual and emotional well-being. It can lead to feelings of frustration,shame and a strain on intimate relationships.

2. Secondary Vaginismus: Secondary Vaginismus refers to the onset of Vaginismus after a period of pain-free sexual intercourse or vaginal penetration. It can develop due to various reasons, including medical conditions, childbirth, trauma, or relationship issues. Secondary Vaginismus can occur after a person has had a satisfying sexual relationship and is often associated with specific triggers or events that cause the involuntary muscle contractions.

SIGNS AND SYMPTOMS OF VAGINISMUS.

The signs and symptoms of vaginismus can vary from person to person, but common indicators of the condition include:

1. Involuntary muscle spasms: The primary symptom of vaginismus is the involuntary tightening or spasming of the pelvic floor muscles, specifically those surrounding the vagina. These spasms can make it difficult or impossible to insert anything into the vagina, leading to pain or discomfort. Normally, these muscles are under voluntary control, meaning we can consciously relax or contract them as needed. However, in individuals with vaginismus, these muscles contract involuntarily and uncontrollably. These spasms can be triggered by the anticipation or attempt of vaginal penetration, such as during sexual intercourse or the insertion of tampons. The muscles tighten and contract, creating a barrier that makes it difficult or impossible for anything to enter the vagina.

2. Pain or discomfort during penetration: Individuals with vaginismus often experience pain or discomfort during attempted vaginal penetration. This can include pain during sexual intercourse, the insertion of tampons, or even during a pelvic exam.

3. Fear or anxiety related to penetration: Due to the pain and discomfort associated with vaginismus, individuals may develop a fear or anxiety surrounding any form of vaginal penetration. This fear can further contribute to muscle tension and spasms, creating a cycle of pain and anxiety.

4. Difficulty with gynecological exams: Difficulty with gynecological exams is a common sign and symptom of vaginismus. When individuals with vaginismus attempt to undergo a gynecological exam, they may experience intense muscle spasms and tightening of the pelvic floor muscles. These spasms can make it extremely uncomfortable or even impossible for a healthcare provider to insert a speculum or perform a thorough examination of the vagina. The fear and anxiety associated with vaginismus can further exacerbate the muscle spasms during gynecological exams. The anticipation of pain or discomfort can trigger a protective response in the body, causing the pelvic floor muscles to tighten involuntarily. As a result, individuals with vaginismus may find it challenging to receive necessary gynecological care, such as Pap smears, pelvic exams, or other procedures. This difficulty can lead to delayed or inadequate medical attention, which may have implications for overall reproductive health.

5. Avoidance of sexual activity: One of the key signs and symptoms of vaginismus is an avoidance of sexual activity. This avoidance can manifest in various ways, such as reluctance or fear of attempting penetration, discomfort or pain during attempts at penetration, or a complete avoidance of any sexual activity altogether. The fear and anticipation of pain or discomfort can create a cycle of anxiety and avoidance, making it challenging for individuals with vaginismus to engage in sexual activities.

It is important to note that the avoidance of sexual activity is not a conscious choice but rather a protective response of the body. The involuntary muscle contractions associated with vaginismus occur as a reflexive response triggered by the fear, anxiety, or anticipation of pain during any form of vaginal penetration. Individuals with vaginismus may avoid sexual activity altogether due to the pain and discomfort they experience. This can strain relationships and lead to feelings of frustration, guilt, or shame.

COMMON MISCONCEPTIONS ABOUT VAGINISMUS.

There are several common misconceptions surrounding vaginismus, which can contribute to misunderstandings and stigma surrounding this condition. It's important to address these misconceptions to promote accurate information and support for individuals experiencing vaginismus. Here are some of the common misconceptions:

1. Vaginismus is a rare condition: Vaginismus is more common than many people realize. While exact prevalence rates are difficult to determine due to underreporting and misdiagnosis, it is estimated that vaginismus affects a significant number of individuals. However, due to the sensitive nature of the condition, many people may not openly discuss it, leading to the misconception that it is rare.

2. Vaginismus is purely a physical problem: While vaginismus is characterized by involuntary muscle spasms in the pelvic floor muscles, it is not solely a physical issue. Psychological factors, such as anxiety, fear, trauma, or negative experiences related to sex, can contribute to the development or exacerbation of vaginismus. It is a complex condition that often requires a multidimensional approach to treatment, addressing both physical and psychological aspects.

3. Vaginismus is caused by a lack of arousal or desire: Vaginismus is not caused by a lack of sexual arousal or desire. It is a condition characterized by involuntary muscle spasms that occur regardless of a person's level of arousal or desire. It is important to understand that vaginismus is a physical response, and the inability to engage in vaginal penetration is not due to a lack of interest or attraction.

4. Vaginismus can be easily overcome by "just relaxing": Telling someone with vaginismus to "just relax" is not helpful and oversimplifies the condition. Vaginismus is not a conscious choice or something that can be easily controlled. It often requires specialized treatment, such as pelvic floor physical therapy, counseling, or other interventions, to address the underlying causes and help individuals manage and overcome the involuntary muscle spasms.

5. Vaginismus is untreatable or incurable: Vaginismus is a treatable condition, and many individuals find relief and improvement with appropriate interventions. Treatment approaches may vary depending on the individual, but options such as pelvic floor physical therapy, counseling, gradual desensitization, and the use of vaginal dilators have been effective for many people. With patience, support, and the right treatment, individuals with vaginismus can experience significant improvement in their symptoms and quality of life.

6. Vaginismus only affects cisgender women: While vaginismus is commonly associated with cisgender women, it can also affect transgender individuals and individuals assigned male at birth. Anyone with a vagina can potentially experience vaginismus, regardless of their gender identity.

CHAPTER 2

PREVENTION AND TREATMENT OPTIONS FOR VAGINISMUS.

Different Ways To Prevent Vaginismus

Vaginismus is a complex condition that can have both physical and psychological causes, making it challenging to prevent entirely. However, there are some steps individuals can take to promote pelvic health and potentially reduce the risk of developing vaginismus. Here are some preventive measures that may be beneficial:

1. Education and awareness: Educating oneself about sexual health, anatomy, and healthy sexual practices can be helpful in promoting a positive and informed approach to sexuality. Understanding the normal range of sexual experiences and knowing that pain or discomfort during penetration is not normal can help individuals seek appropriate support and treatment if needed.

2. Open communication:

Establishing open and honest communication with sexual partners is crucial. Discussing desires, boundaries, and any concerns related to sexual activities can help create a safe and supportive environment. This can also help identify and address any potential issues early on, reducing the risk of developing vaginismus due to unresolved emotional or relationship factors.

3. Gradual exploration and relaxation techniques:

Engaging in gradual exploration

of one's own body and becoming comfortable with self-touch can help individuals develop a positive relationship with their own sexuality. This can involve self-exploration, using lubrication, and practicing relaxation techniques, such as deep breathing or mindfulness exercises, to promote relaxation and reduce muscle tension.

4. Seeking professional guidance: If individuals have concerns or difficulties related to sexual health or experiencing pain or discomfort during penetration, it is important to seek professional guidance. Consulting with a healthcare provider, such as a gynecologist or a sex therapist, can help identify any underlying physical or psychological factors and provide appropriate guidance and treatment options.

5. Addressing trauma or negative experiences:

Traumatic experiences, such as sexual abuse or assault, can contribute to the development of vaginismus. Seeking therapy or counseling to address and process any past trauma can be beneficial in preventing or managing vaginismus. It is important to create a safe and supportive environment to heal from any past negative experiences.

6. Pelvic floor exercises:

Engaging in regular pelvic floor exercises, also known as Kegel exercises, can help strengthen and maintain the pelvic floor muscles. Strong pelvic floor muscles can contribute to overall pelvic health and potentially reduce the risk of muscle spasms associated with vaginismus. However, it is important to note that excessive or incorrect pelvic floor exercises can also contribute to muscle tension, so it is advisable to consult with a healthcare professional for guidance on proper technique and frequency.

TREATMENT OPTIONS FOR VAGINISMUS.

There are several treatment options available for vaginismus, and the most effective approach may vary depending on the individual's specific needs and circumstances. It's important to consult with a healthcare professional, such as a gynecologist or a sex therapist, to determine the most suitable treatment plan. Here are some common treatment options for vaginismus:

1. Pelvic floor physical therapy: Pelvic floor physical therapy involves working with a specialized physical therapist who can help identify and address any muscle imbalances or tension in the pelvic floor muscles. The therapist may use techniques such as manual therapy, biofeedback, and exercises to help relax and strengthen the pelvic floor muscles. This approach can be particularly beneficial for individuals with vaginismus caused by physical factors.

2. Gradual desensitization: Gradual desensitization involves a step-by-step approach to gradually introduce vaginal penetration. This can be done using vaginal dilators or other similar devices of increasing sizes. The individual starts with the smallest dilator and gradually progresses to larger sizes as they become more comfortable. This technique helps desensitize the body to penetration and allows the individual to regain control over their pelvic muscles.

3. Cognitive-behavioral therapy (CBT): CBT is a form of therapy that focuses on identifying and changing negative thought patterns and behaviors. In the context of vaginismus, CBT can help individuals address any underlying anxiety, fear, or negative beliefs related to sex and penetration. It can also provide coping strategies and relaxation techniques to manage the physical and emotional aspects of vaginismus.

4. Counseling or sex therapy: Counseling or sex therapy can be beneficial for individuals with vaginismus, especially if there are underlying psychological factors contributing to the condition. A therapist can provide a safe and supportive environment to explore any emotional or relationship issues, address past trauma, and develop strategies to improve sexual well-being.

5. Medications: In some cases, healthcare professionals may prescribe medications to help manage the symptoms of vaginismus. These medications may include muscle relaxants, topical anesthetics, or low-dose antidepressants. Medications are typically used in conjunction with other treatment approaches and are tailored to the individual's specific needs.

6. Surgical options: Surgical options for vaginismus are considered as a last resort and are typically only pursued after other conservative treatment approaches have been exhausted. Surgical options are generally not considered as a primary treatment for vaginismus. Vaginismus is primarily a condition characterized by involuntary muscle spasms in the pelvic floor muscles, and surgical interventions typically do not directly address the underlying muscle tension or psychological factors associated with vaginismus. However, in rare cases where other treatment options have been unsuccessful or if there are specific anatomical abnormalities contributing to the condition, surgical interventions may be considered as a last resort. It's important to note that the decision to pursue surgical options should be made in consultation with a healthcare professional who specializes in sexual health and has experience with vaginismus. There are a few surgical procedures for vaginismus. These procedures aim to address physical factors that may contribute to the condition. However, it's important to emphasize that the evidence supporting the effectiveness of these surgical interventions is limited, and their use is controversial.

Here are a few surgical options that have been explored:

1. Vestibulectomy:

Vestibulectomy is a surgical procedure that involves the removal of the sensitive tissue at the entrance of the vagina, known as the vestibule. This procedure aims to reduce pain and discomfort during penetration by removing the hypersensitive tissue. However, it is important to note that this procedure does not directly address the muscle spasms associated with vaginismus and may not be effective for all individuals.

2. Botox injections: Botox injections have been used in some cases to temporarily paralyze the pelvic floor muscles, thereby reducing muscle spasms. The injections are typically administered directly into the pelvic floor muscles under anesthesia. However, the effects of Botox injections are temporary, and the procedure may need to be repeated periodically.

3. Hymenectomy: In cases where an imperforate hymen or a thick hymen is contributing to the muscle spasms and pain associated with vaginismus, a hymenectomy may be considered. This surgical procedure involves the removal or modification of the hymen to allow for pain-free penetration. However, it's important to note that hymenectomy alone may not address the underlying muscle tension or psychological factors associated with vaginismus.

CHAPTER 3

SELF CARE TECHNIQUES.

Self-care techniques can be helpful for individuals with vaginismus to manage symptoms, promote relaxation, and support overall well-being. Here are some self-care techniques that may be beneficial:

1. Deep breathing exercises: Deep breathing can help promote relaxation and reduce muscle tension. Practice slow, full breaths, breathing in profoundly through your nose and breathing out leisurely through your mouth. Focus on relaxing your pelvic floor muscles as you breathe out.

2. Pelvic relaxation exercises: Engage in regular pelvic relaxation exercises to help release tension in the pelvic floor muscles. Lie down in a comfortable position and consciously relax your pelvic floor muscles. You can visualize the muscles softening and releasing any tension. Combine this with deep breathing for enhanced relaxation.

3. Warm baths or sitz baths: Soaking in a warm bath or taking sitz baths (sitting in a shallow basin of warm water) can help relax the pelvic floor muscles and provide soothing relief. Adding Epsom salts or essential oils to the bathwater may enhance relaxation.

4. Gentle stretching: Gentle stretching exercises, such as yoga or Pilates, can help improve flexibility and release tension in the body, including the pelvic floor muscles. Focus on gentle stretches that target the hips, lower back, and pelvic area.

5. Stress management techniques: Stress and anxiety can exacerbate vaginismus symptoms. Engage in stress management techniques that work for you, such as meditation, mindfulness, journaling, or engaging in hobbies or activities that bring you joy and relaxation.

6. Lubrication: Using a water-based lubricant during sexual activities or when attempting penetration can help reduce friction and discomfort. Choose a lubricant that is free from irritants and compatible with your body.

NOTE: Self-care techniques are not a substitute for professional treatment.

CHAPTER 4.

COPING STRATEGIES FOR VAGINISMUS.

Coping strategies and emotional support are crucial for individuals with vaginismus as they navigate the challenges and emotions associated with the condition. Here are some coping strategies and sources of emotional support that can be helpful:

1. Communicate with your partner: Open and honest communication with your partner is essential. Share your feelings, fears, and concerns about vaginismus. Educate them about the condition and involve them in your treatment journey. A supportive and understanding partner can provide emotional support, patience, and reassurance.

2. Explore non-penetrative intimacy: Focus on non-penetrative sexual activities that bring pleasure and intimacy to your relationship. Engage in activities such as kissing, cuddling, caressing or massage can help maintain a connection with your partner and foster intimacy while you work on managing vaginismus.

3. Education and self-awareness: Educate yourself about vaginismus to gain a better understanding of the condition. This can help normalize your experiences and reduce feelings of isolation. Learn about the causes, symptoms, and available treatment options. Being all around informed can enable you to settle on informed conclusions about your consideration.

4. Seek professional support:
Reach out to healthcare professionals who specialize in sexual health or have experience with vaginismus. They can provide guidance, support, and appropriate treatment options. A gynecologist, sex therapist, or pelvic floor physical therapist can offer valuable insights and help you develop a personalized treatment plan.

5. Join support groups:
Consider joining support groups or online communities where

you can connect with others who have similar experiences. Sharing your thoughts, concerns, and successes with individuals who understand can provide validation, support, and a sense of belonging. Hearing others' stories and learning from their coping strategies can be empowering.

6. Practice self-empathy: Be thoughtful and delicate with yourself. Vaginismus is not your fault, and it does not define your worth or desirability. Practice self-compassion by acknowledging your emotions, accepting yourself as you are, and treating yourself with love and understanding. Celebrate small victories and be patient with the healing process.

7. Seek therapy or counseling: Consider individual therapy or couples therapy with a therapist who specializes in sexual health. Therapy can provide a safe space to explore and address any emotional or psychological factors contributing to vaginismus. It can help you develop coping strategies, manage anxiety, and improve overall well-being.

8. Practice stress management techniques: Stress can exacerbate vaginismus symptoms. Engage in stress management techniques that work for you, such as deep breathing, meditation, yoga, or engaging in hobbies that bring you joy and relaxation. Focus on taking care of oneself and set aside a few minutes for exercises that help you loosen up and decrease pressure.

CONCLUSION.

In conclusion, dealing with vaginismus can be a challenging and complex journey, but with the right support and resources, individuals can find relief and improve their quality of life. Vaginismus is a condition characterized by involuntary muscle spasms in the pelvic floor muscles, specifically the muscles around the vagina. It can cause pain, discomfort, and difficulty with vaginal penetration, impacting sexual activities, gynecological exams, and overall well-being. It is important to understand that vaginismus is not a reflection of a person's worth or desirability. It is a medical condition that can have both physical and psychological causes. Seeking professional help from healthcare providers who specialize in sexual health, such as gynecologists, sex therapists, or pelvic floor physical therapists, is crucial for accurate diagnosis and appropriate treatment. It is also important to note that treatment for vaginismus is highly individualized, and what works for one person may not work for another. Tolerance, ingenuity, and open correspondence with medical care experts are critical. In addition to professional treatment, self-care techniques and coping strategies play a vital role in managing vaginismus. Engaging in relaxation exercises, stress management techniques, joining support groups, and practicing self-compassion can help individuals cope with the emotional and physical challenges of vaginismus. It is essential to remember that vaginismus is a treatable condition, and many individuals find relief and improvement with appropriate interventions. While the journey may have its ups and downs, with time, support, and a comprehensive approach, individuals can overcome vaginismus and reclaim their sexual well-being.